Copyright ©2020 ARNOLD KUNTZ PH.D

CONTENTS

INTRODUCTION

Lyme disease is a bacterial infection caused by various species of Borrelia. These are all spirochaetes (spiral-shaped bacteria), that can in certain circumstances change into a cyst-like form that is very hard to detect. The disease is in most cases caught when a juvenile tick about the size of a sesame seed latches onto your skin with its legs and pushes its chelicerae (cutting tools) and feeding tube through your skin. It also secretes a numbing agent to help it avoid detection. It stays attached for up to two days as it drinks a huge amount of blood in comparison to its body size. The longer it stays attached, the greater your chances of getting Lyme disease, assuming of course that the tick is one that has Lyme disease itself. Most ticks do not. So if you are bitten by a tick, the chance of getting Lyme could be anywhere between 1-30%, but in the UK the percentage chance of getting Lyme is normally on the lower end of this range. Ticks that carry Lyme disease are found in most regions of the UK, especially Scotland and the south of England. Those that intend to infect you are found at the top of long grasses from where they can attach to your clothing or bare legs. They like wet temperate conditions and will be more prevalent after wet weather. In hot, dry conditions, they are more likely to be found on logs or in leaf litter.

HOW CAN LYME DISEASE AFFECT YOUR BODY?

Lyme disease is able to affect your immune system in a number of ways, specifically causing three major effects, including:

Lowered immunity - this puts you at risk of further different types of infection that may have been transmitted with the original tick bite. These include babesiosis, bartonella, ehrlichiosis, rickettsia, mycoplasma, and chlamydia. Many of these display flu-like symptoms, and it is often difficult to tell these infections apart. A number of these diseases also have the potential to cause long term complications.

Autoimmunity - this is where your immune system starts attacking your own tissues. Examples include multiple sclerosis and rheumatoid arthritis, which are associated with Lyme disease.

Inflammation - this plays a role in virtually all diseases that affect us. More specifically with Lyme, there are associations with Parkinson's, Alzheimer's, and Motor Neuron disease, reflecting the extent to which Lyme disease attacks the central nervous system.

SYMPTOMS OF LYME DISEASE

After an infected tick has detached from your skin and the bacteria have entered your bloodstream, it may take up to a month to develop any symptoms. These can include in somewhere between 30-70% of cases a distinctive bull's eye rash which is known as 'erythema migrans', meaning a rash that can move about the body. Other acute symptoms can include;

Sweats and chills

Headaches and neck pain

Muscle and joint aches

Insomnia

If the infection is left untreated or antibiotic treatment fails, then it is possible to get longer-term chronic symptoms, which include;

Fatigue

Depression, anxiety, and cognitive defects

Persistent muscle and joint aches

Tingling extremities

Cardiac problems such as heart block and arrhythmias

Because Lyme disease causes big changes to your immune system, persistent chronic Lyme infection can increase your chances of contracting Multiple Sclerosis, Rheumatoid Arthritis, and certain dementias.

LYME INFLAMMATION DIET

Dietary steps to improve symptoms

Step 1
Remove inflammatory foods, including;

All processed foods, which strongly associated with inflammation

Processed cooking oils which are also responsible for increased inflammation

Foods high in sugars that trigger inflammatory responses, partially due to changes in your gut flora

Gluten-containing foods may also cause inflammation in some people via increased intestinal permeability, which allows foreign proteins to enter the bloodstream triggering an immune response.

Step 2
Include anti-inflammatory foods.

Meat and fish that is well reared or caught, such as those that have organic certification.

Daily portions of vegetables. Vegetables with a higher glycaemic index such as potatoes should be moderated as a high blood sugar level can impair the immune response to Lyme disease.

Healthy oils, nuts, and seeds contain fats that are anti-inflammatory as well as important anti-inflammatory vitamins and minerals. The healthy oils include olive oil, coconut oil, cod liver oil, butter, and lard. Nuts and seeds should be in their natural state and not coated with sunflower oil or other processed oils.

Some grains may be OK, but many people with Lyme and imbalanced gut flora will struggle to eat large portions of lentils, beans, or other grain-based foods.

Step 3
Support your glutathione and Nrf2 detoxification systems by eating foods that contain the nutrients that help build your glutathione system. These include;

The amino acids that help build the glutathione system, the most important of which is gelatin found in particular in the offcuts of meat that people eschew for muscle meats nowadays. Gelatin is found in particular in connective tissues that connect our skeleton together. Bone broth and brawn are two options that are relatively easy to obtain from your local butchers. For vegans without strict adherence to veganism, jelly and marshmallow are options. For strict vegans, beans, legumes, nuts, and seeds offer the best glycine containing possibilities. Pumpkin seeds contain particularly good amounts.

The mineral selenium is a key component of your glutathione system and can be obtained from Brazil nuts, most fish and seafood, as well as chicken and eggs.

Many vegetables, especially the leafy greens and onion family contain compounds that help boost the glutathione system.

Eating foods that contain nutrients that boost your Nrf2 anti-oxidant system, including;

Berries of all types, chocolate, red wine, and green tea, which all contain compounds that boost the Nrf2 system. Too many of these compounds, however, has been shown to reverse the benefits to your Nrf2 system, so keep your intake of these foods to regular, moderate portion sizes.

Step 4
Keep your immune system generally supported by getting enough vitamin D, either through sunshine or vitamin D containing foods such as cod liver oil, liver, or butter.

RECEPIES

CAJUN SPICE MIX

Ingredients

2 teaspoons salt

2 teaspoons garlic powder

2 ½ teaspoons paprika

1 teaspoon ground black pepper

1 teaspoon onion powder

1 teaspoon cayenne pepper

1 ¼ teaspoons dried oregano

1 ¼ teaspoons dried thyme

½ teaspoon red pepper flakes

Directions

STEP 1

Stir together salt, garlic powder, paprika, black pepper, onion powder, cayenne pepper, oregano, thyme, and red pepper flakes until evenly blended. Store in an airtight container.

Nutrition Facts Per Serving:
6 calories; protein 0.2g 1% DV; carbohydrates 1.2g; fat 0.1g; cholesterol mg; sodium 388.2mg 16% DV.

HOMEMADE POULTRY SEASONING

Ingredients

2 teaspoons ground dried sage

1 ½ teaspoons ground dried thyme

1 teaspoon ground dried marjoram

¾ teaspoon ground dried rosemary

½ teaspoon ground nutmeg

½ teaspoon finely ground black pepper

Directions

STEP 1

Combine sage, thyme, marjoram, rosemary, nutmeg, and black pepper in sealable container; store with your other spices until needed.

Nutrition Facts Per Serving:
1 calories; proteing; carbohydrates 0.2g; fatg; cholesterolmg; sodium 0.1mg.

THE FAMOUS SEAFOOD SEASONING RECIPE

Ingredients

6 ⅓ tablespoons salt

3 ⅔ tablespoons ground celery seed

2 ½ teaspoons dry mustard powder

2 ½ teaspoons red pepper flakes, ground

1 ½ teaspoons ground black pepper

1 ½ teaspoons ground bay leaves

1 ½ teaspoons paprika

1 teaspoon ground cloves

1 teaspoon ground allspice

1 teaspoon ground ginger

¾ teaspoon ground cardamom

½ teaspoon ground cinnamon

Directions
Step 1
Mix the salt, celery seed, dry mustard powder, red

pepper, black pepper, bay leaves, paprika, cloves, allspice, ginger, cardamom, and cinnamon together in a bowl until thoroughly combined. Store in an airtight container.

Nutrition Facts Per Serving:
1 calories; proteing; carbohydrates 0.1g; fat 0.1g; cholesterolmg; sodium 245.7mg 10% DV.

GREAT STEAK SEASONING

Ingredients

2 tablespoons coarse-ground black pepper

2 tablespoons paprika

1 tablespoon kosher salt

1 tablespoon granulated garlic

1 tablespoon dill seed

1 tablespoon ground coriander

1 tablespoon red pepper flakes

Directions

Step 1

Grind black pepper, paprika, kosher salt, granulated garlic, dill seed, coriander seed, and red pepper flakes together with a mortar and pestle or in a spice grinder. Store in a sealed glass container.

Nutrition Facts Per Serving:

8 calories; protein 0.4g 1% DV; carbohydrates 1.7g 1% DV; fat 0.3g; cholesterolmg; sodium 288.9mg 12% DV.

AUTHENTIC CANADIAN STEAK SPICE, EH?

Ingredients

2 tablespoons white peppercorns

1 tablespoon coriander seed

2 teaspoons dill seed

2 teaspoons mustard seed

1 teaspoon red pepper flakes

2 tablespoons dried minced garlic

2 tablespoons kosher salt

Directions

Step 1

Place white peppercorns into a mini food processor or spice grinder; pulse several times. Add coriander seed, dill seed, mustard seed, and red pepper flakes to food processor; pulse until seeds are broken into a coarse mixture.

Step 2

Transfer spice mixture to a small bowl; stir in garlic and kosher salt. Store mixture in an airtight glass container;

shake before using.

Nutrition Facts Per Serving:
7 calories; protein 0.3g 1% DV; carbohydrates 1.3g; fat 0.2g; cholesterolmg; sodium 480.4mg 19% DV.

INSALATA CAPRESE II

Ingredients

4 large ripe tomatoes, sliced 1/4 inch thick

1 pound fresh mozzarella cheese, sliced 1/4 inch thick

⅓ cup fresh basil leaves

3 tablespoons extra virgin olive oil

Fine sea salt to taste

Freshly ground black pepper to taste

Directions

Step 1

On a large platter, alternate and overlap the tomato slices, mozzarella cheese slices, and basil leaves. Drizzle with olive oil. Season with sea salt and pepper.

Nutrition Facts Per Serving:

311 calories; protein 17.9g 36% DV; carbohydrates 6.6g 2% DV; fat 23.9g 37% DV; cholesterol 59.8mg 20% DV; sodium 627.3mg 25% DV.

INSALATA CAPRESE I

Ingredients

4 ripe tomatoes, cut into wedges

14 ounces fresh mozzarella cheese, diced

1 red onion, sliced

⅓ Cup extra virgin olive oil

⅓ Cup balsamic vinegar

¼ cup chopped fresh basil

Salt and pepper to taste

Directions

STEP 1

In a large bowl, combine the tomatoes, cheese, onion, oil, vinegar, basil, and salt and pepper to taste. Toss and chill for 1 hour. Serve on large platter.

Nutrition Facts Per Serving:

498 calories; protein 19.3g 39% DV; carbohydrates 12.7g 4% DV; fat 40.3g 62% DV; cholesterol 77.9mg 26% DV; sodium 154.2mg 6% DV.

CAPRESE SALAD

Ingredients

8 ounces fresh mozzarella cheese, cubed

1 (10 ounce) basket cherry tomatoes

3 tablespoons torn fresh basil leaves

1 tablespoon olive oil

Salt and pepper to taste

Directions

STEP 1

Toss together the mozzarella, cherry tomatoes, basil, and olive oil in a large bowl. Season with salt and pepper.

Nutrition Facts Per Serving:
189 calories; protein 14.4g 29% DV; carbohydrates 4.9g 2% DV; fat 12.6g 20% DV; cholesterol 36.3mg 12% DV; sodium 357.5mg 14% DV.

THE BEST CAPRESE SALAD

Ingredients

3 large heirloom tomatoes, sliced, or to taste

1 (16 ounce) package fresh mozzarella cheese, sliced

½ cup fresh basil leaves

3 tablespoons extra-virgin olive oil

Salt and ground black pepper to taste

Directions

Step 1

Arrange tomato slices, mozzarella slices, and basil leaves on a serving plate, alternating between them. Drizzle with olive oil and sprinkle with salt and pepper.

Nutrition Facts Per Serving:

405 calories; protein 28.9g 58% DV; carbohydrates 8.6g 3% DV; fat 28.5g 44% DV; cholesterol 72.6mg 24% DV; sodium 748.4mg 30% DV.

SIMPLE CAPRESE SALAD

Ingredients

1 (12 ounce) jar roasted red peppers, drained

16 slices fresh mozzarella cheese

16 thick slices ripe slicing tomato

32 leaves fresh basil

Olive oil

1 pinch ground black pepper to taste

1 (4 ounce) can sliced black olives, drained

Directions

STEP 1

Cut roasted red peppers into 16 large pieces. Starting at the edge of a serving platter, place a slice of tomato, a basil leaf, a slice of mozzarella cheese, a piece of roasted pepper, and another basil leaf. Continue in that pattern, forming a spiral from the outside in, until all the ingredients have been arranged; salad should end in the center of the platter. Drizzle the salad with olive oil and sprinkle with black pepper and black olives.

Nutrition Facts Per Serving:
311 calories; protein 15.2g 30% DV; carbohydrates 9.1g 3% DV; fat 23.2g 36% DV; cholesterol 59.4mg 20% DV; sodium 478.8mg 19% DV.

GRILLED ASPARAGUS

Ingredients

1 pound fresh asparagus spears, trimmed

1 tablespoon olive oil

Salt and pepper to taste

Directions

Step 1

Preheat grill for high heat.

Step 2

Lightly coat the asparagus spears with olive oil. Season with salt and pepper to taste.

STEP 3

Grill over high heat for 2 to 3 minutes, or to desired tenderness.

Nutrition Facts Per Serving:
53 calories; protein 2.5g 5% DV; carbohydrates 4.4g 1% DV; fat 3.5g 5% DV; cholesterolmg; sodium 2.3mg.

GRILLED SOY-SESAME ASPARAGUS

Ingredients

1 tablespoon toasted sesame oil

1 tablespoon soy sauce

3 cloves garlic, minced

1 teaspoon brown sugar

1 ½ pounds fresh asparagus, trimmed

2 tablespoons toasted sesame seeds

Directions

Step 1

Preheat grill for high heat.

Step 2

In a bowl, mix sesame oil, soy sauce, garlic, and brown sugar. Place asparagus in the bowl, and toss to coat.

Step 3

Lightly oil a fine-mesh grill grate. Place asparagus on grate, and cook 8 minutes, until tender but firm. Garnish with sesame seeds to serve.

Nutrition Facts Per Serving:

100 calories; protein 4.9g 10% DV; carbohydrates 9.8g 3% DV; fat 5.9g 9% DV; cholesterolmg; sodium

230.1mg 9% DV.

THE BEST STEAMED ASPARAGUS

Ingredients

1 pound fresh asparagus spears, trimmed

¼ cup white wine

2 tablespoons butter

Directions

Step 1

Place asparagus in a microwave-safe dish. Pour in wine, and dot with pieces of butter.

STEP 2

Cover loosely, and cook in the microwave on High for 3 minutes, or until bright green and tender. Allow the dish to stand 5 minutes before serving.

Nutrition Facts Per Serving:
86 calories; protein 2.6g 5% DV; carbohydrates 4.8g 2% DV; fat 5.9g 9% DV; cholesterol 15.3mg 5% DV; sodium 43.9mg 2% DV.

ROASTED ASPARAGUS AND GARLIC

Ingredients

12 cloves garlic

2 tablespoons olive oil

¼ cup white wine

3 cups diagonally sliced asparagus

6 sprigs fresh thyme

Directions

Step 1

Preheat the oven to 350 degrees F (175 degrees C).

STEP 2

Tear off 6 large pieces of foil. Divide garlic, olive oil, wine, asparagus, and thyme and arrange them on each piece of foil. Fold over each foil packet to seal. Place the packets on a baking sheet and roast for 20 to 25 minutes until the asparagus is tender, but still a little crisp. Carefully open packets and serve asparagus with juices poured on top.

Nutrition Facts Per Serving:
72 calories; protein 1.9g 4% DV; carbohydrates 5.1g 2% DV; fat 4.6g 7% DV; cholesterolmg; sodium 3.2mg.

AWESOMELY EASY SESAME ASPARAGUS

Ingredients

1 bunch fresh asparagus, trimmed

1 tablespoon olive oil

2 tablespoons black sesame seeds, lightly toasted

Kosher salt to taste

Directions

Step 1

Fill a large saucepan with 1/2 inch of water and bring to a boil. Cook asparagus until tender-crisp, about 5 minutes. Drain, then rinse with cold water. Return pan to the stove over medium heat, pour in oil, and swirl around pan. Shake excess water off of the asparagus, and toss in oil with sesame seeds, and salt to reheat.

Nutrition Facts Per Serving:

78 calories; protein 3.3g 7% DV; carbohydrates 5.5g 2% DV; fat 5.7g 9% DV; cholesterolmg; sodium 102.8mg 4% DV.

EASY HERB-ROASTED TURKEY

Ingredients

1 (12 pound) whole turkey

¾ cup olive oil

2 tablespoons garlic powder

2 teaspoons dried basil

1 teaspoon ground sage

1 teaspoon salt

½ teaspoon black pepper

2 cups water

Directions

STEP 1

Preheat oven to 325 degrees F (165 degrees C). Clean turkey (discard giblets and organs), and place in a roasting pan with a lid.

STEP 2

In a small bowl, combine olive oil, garlic powder, dried basil, ground sage, salt, and black pepper. Using a basting brush, apply the mixture to the outside of the uncooked turkey. Pour water into the bottom of the roasting pan, and cover.

STEP 3

Bake for 3 to 3 1/2 hours, or until the internal temperature of the thickest part of the thigh measures 180 degrees F (82 degrees C). Remove bird from oven, and allow to stand for about 30 minutes before carving.

Nutrition Facts Per Serving:
597 calories; protein 68.2g 136% DV; carbohydrates 0.9g; fat 33.7g 52% DV; cholesterol 198.3mg 66% DV; sodium 311.3mg 13% DV.

ROSEMARY ROASTED TURKEY

Ingredients

¾ cup olive oil

3 tablespoons minced garlic

2 tablespoons chopped fresh rosemary

1 tablespoon chopped fresh basil

1 tablespoon Italian seasoning

1 teaspoon ground black pepper

Salt to taste

1 (12 pound) whole turkey

Directions
Step 1
Preheat oven to 325 degrees F (165 degrees C).

STEP 2

In a small bowl, mix the olive oil, garlic, rosemary, basil, Italian seasoning, black pepper and salt. Set aside.

STEP 3

Wash the turkey inside and out; pat dry. Remove any large fat deposits. Loosen the skin from the breast. This is done by slowly working your fingers between the breast and the skin. Work it loose to the end of the drumstick, being careful not to tear the skin.

STEP 4

Using your hand, spread a generous amount of the rosemary mixture under the breast skin and down the thigh and leg. Rub the remainder of the rosemary mixture over the outside of the breast. Use toothpicks to seal skin over any exposed breast meat.

Step 5

Place the turkey on a rack in a roasting pan. Add about 1/4 inch of water to the bottom of the pan. Roast in the preheated oven 3 to 4 hours, or until the internal temperature of the bird reaches 180 degrees F (80 degrees C).

Nutrition Facts Per Serving:

597 calories; protein 68.1g 136% DV; carbohydrates 0.8g; fat 33.7g 52% DV; cholesterol 198.3mg 66% DV; sodium 165.1mg 7% DV.

SMOKED TURKEY

Ingredients

1 (12 pound) whole turkey, neck and giblets removed

1 (20 pound) bag high quality charcoal briquettes

Hickory chips or chunks

Directions

STEP 1

Place the charcoal into the bottom pan of the smoker. Light the coals and wait for the temperature of the smoker to come to 240 degrees F (115 degrees C). Lightly oil grate.

Step 2

Rinse turkey under cold water, and pat dry. Place hickory chips into a pan with water to cover.

Step 3

Place turkey onto the prepared grate. Add 2 handfuls damp chips at start of cooking, then a handful every couple of hours during the cooking process. Leave the lid on - DO NOT keep looking at the turkey, or you will let the heat out! Continue smoking until the internal temperature of the turkey reaches 165 degrees F (74 degrees C), or keep going until the coals die out.

Nutrition Facts Per Serving:

447 calories; protein 60.4g 121% DV; carbohydratesg; fat 20.9g 32% DV; cholesterol 176.3mg 59% DV; sodium 146.2mg 6% DV.

THE GREATEST GRILLED TURKEY

Ingredients

12 pounds whole turkey

1 tablespoon vegetable oil

1 teaspoon Italian seasoning

Salt and pepper to taste

Directions

STEP 1

Prepare an outdoor grill for indirect medium-high heat.

STEP 2

Rinse turkey and pat dry. Turn wings back to hold neck skin in place. Return legs to tucked position. Brush turkey with oil. Season inside and out with Italian seasonings, salt, and pepper.

STEP 3

Place turkey, breast side up, on a metal grate inside a large roasting pan. Arrange pan on the prepared grill. Grill 2 to 3 hours, to an internal thigh temperature of 180 degrees F (85 degrees C). Remove turkey from grill and let stand 15 minutes before carving.

Nutrition Facts Per Serving:
460 calories; protein 61.2g 123% DV; carbohydrates 0.1g; fat 22g 34% DV; cholesterol 178.7mg 60% DV; sodium 148.2mg 6% DV.

SIMPLE CLASSIC ROASTED TURKEY

Ingredients

1 (10 pound) whole turkey, neck and giblets optional

Salt and ground black pepper to taste

⅓ Cup water, or as needed

Directions

Step 1

Preheat oven to 275 degrees F (135 degrees C).

Step 2

Season turkey with salt and pepper and place, breast-side down, in a roaster; add neck and giblets. Pour water into pan.

Step 3

Bake in the preheated oven, basting as needed, until no longer pink at the bone and the juices run clear, about 6 hours. An instant-read thermometer inserted into the thickest part of the thigh should read 165 degrees F (74 degrees C). Continue to roast until meat falls off the bone if desired.

Nutrition Facts Per Serving:

567 calories; protein 76.6g 153% DV; carbohydratesg; fat 26.5g 41% DV; cholesterol 223.5mg 75% DV; sodium

185.6mg 7% DV.

MARINATED GRILLED SHRIMP

Ingredients

3 cloves garlic, minced

⅓ Cup olive oil

¼ cup tomato sauce

2 tablespoons red wine vinegar

2 tablespoons chopped fresh basil

½ teaspoon salt

¼ teaspoon cayenne pepper

2 pounds fresh shrimp, peeled and deveined

Skewers

Directions

STEP 1

In a large bowl, stir together the garlic, olive oil, tomato sauce, and red wine vinegar. Season with basil, salt, and cayenne pepper. Add shrimp to the bowl, and stir until evenly coated. Cover, and refrigerate for 30 minutes to 1 hour, stirring once or twice.

Step 2

Preheat grill for medium heat. Thread shrimp onto skewers, piercing once near the tail and once near the head. Discard marinade.

Step 3

Lightly oil grill grate. Cook shrimp on preheated grill for 2 to 3 minutes per side, or until opaque.

Nutrition Facts Per Serving:

273 calories; protein 31g 62% DV; carbohydrates 2.8g 1% DV; fat 14.7g 23% DV; cholesterol 230mg 77% DV; sodium 471.8mg 19% DV.

BIG M'S SPICY LIME GRILLED PRAWNS

Ingredients

48 large tiger prawns, peeled and deveined

4 lime (2" dia)s limes, zested and juiced

4 peppers green chile peppers, seeded and chopped

4 cloves garlic, crushed

1 (2 inch) piece fresh ginger root, chopped

1 medium onion, coarsely chopped

Directions

Step 1

Place the prawns and lime zest in a large, non-metallic bowl. Place the lime juice, chile pepper, garlic, ginger, and onion in a food processor or blender, and process until smooth. You may need to add a little oil to facilitate blending. Pour over the bowl of prawns, and stir to coat. Cover, and refrigerate for 4 hours.

Step 2

Preheat grill for medium-high heat. Thread prawns onto skewers, piercing each first through the tail, and then the head.

Step 3

Brush grill grate with oil. Cook prawns for 5 minutes, turning once, or until opaque.

Nutrition Facts Per Serving:
62 calories; protein 9.8g 20% DV; carbohydrates 5.1g 2% DV; fat 0.6g 1% DV; cholesterol 85.1mg 28% DV; sodium 100mg 4% DV.

HAWAIIAN SHRIMP

Ingredients

2 pounds medium shrimp, peeled and deveined

2 (20 ounce) cans pineapple chunks, juice reserved

½ pound bacon slices, cut into 2 inch pieces

2 large red bell peppers, chopped

½ pound fresh mushrooms, stems removed

2 cups cherry tomatoes

1 cup sweet and sour sauce

Directions
Step 1
Preheat grill for high heat.

Step 2
Thread shrimp, pineapple, bacon, red bell peppers, mushroom caps, and cherry tomatoes on skewers, alternating ingredients. Place in a shallow baking dish. In a small bowl, mix sweet and sour sauce with reserved pineapple juice. Reserve a small amount for basting. Pour remaining sauce over skewers.

Step 3
Lightly oil grill grate. Cook kabobs on preheated grill for 6 to 8 minutes, or until opaque, basting often with reserved sauce.

Nutrition Facts Per Serving:

385 calories; protein 32.4g 65% DV; carbohydrates 47.1g 15% DV; fat 8.1g 12% DV; cholesterol 244mg 81% DV; sodium 714mg 29% DV.

BASIL SHRIMP

Ingredients

2 ½ tablespoons olive oil

¼ cup butter, melted

1 ½ fruit (2-1/8" dia)s lemons, juiced

3 tablespoons Dijon mustard (such as Grey Poupon Country Mustard™)

½ cup minced fresh basil leaves

3 cloves garlic, minced

Salt to taste

White pepper

3 pounds fresh shrimp, peeled and deveined

Directions

Step 1

In a shallow, non-porous dish or bowl, mix together olive oil and melted butter. Stir in lemon juice, mustard, basil, and garlic, and season with salt and white pepper. Add shrimp, and toss to coat. Cover, and refrigerate for 1 hour.

Step 2

Preheat grill to high heat. Remove shrimp from marinade, and thread onto skewers. Discard marinade.

STEP 3

Lightly oil grill grate, and arrange skewers on preheated grill. Cook for 4 minutes, turning once, or until opaque.

Nutrition Facts Per Serving:
206 calories; protein 25g 50% DV; carbohydrates 2.4g 1% DV; fat 10.2g 16% DV; cholesterol 243.9mg 81% DV; sodium 426.4mg 17% DV.

RUM GLAZED GRILLED SHRIMP

Ingredients

¼ cup honey

½ teaspoon lime juice

3 tablespoons spiced rum

½ teaspoon grated orange zest

1 tablespoon orange juice

1 teaspoon grated fresh ginger

1 tablespoon chopped fresh cilantro leaves

¼ teaspoon salt

¼ teaspoon ground black pepper

1 ½ teaspoons cornstarch

20 eaches jumbo shrimp, peeled and deveined

4 eaches (10 inch) skewers

Directions

Step 1

Preheat an outdoor grill for medium heat, and lightly oil the grate.

Step 2

Mix together the honey, lime juice, spiced rum, orange zest, orange juice, ginger, cilantro, salt, black pepper, and cornstarch in a large bowl until the glaze is smooth and the cornstarch is thoroughly blended with the rest of the ingredients. Pour half the glaze into a smaller bowl for basting. Rinse and pat the shrimp dry, and gently stir into the large bowl to thoroughly coat the shrimp with the glaze.

STEP 3

Remove from the glaze, and discard the used glaze. Thread 5 shrimp onto each skewer, and sprinkle with salt and black pepper.

Step 4

Grill the shrimp until bright pink and opaque and the glaze has cooked onto the shrimp, about 4 minutes per side. Baste with additional unused glaze before turning the shrimp over.

Nutrition Facts Per Serving:

232 calories; protein 28.7g 57% DV; carbohydrates 19.1g 6% DV; fat 1.5g 2% DV; cholesterol 266.2mg 89% DV; sodium 452.7mg 18% DV.

FOOLPROOF RIB ROAST

Ingredients

1 (5 pound) standing beef rib roast

2 teaspoons salt

1 teaspoon ground black pepper

1 teaspoon garlic powder

Directions

Step 1

Allow roast to stand at room temperature for at least 1 hour.

Step 2

Preheat the oven to 375 degrees F (190 degrees C). Combine the salt, pepper and garlic powder in a small cup. Place the roast on a rack in a roasting pan so that the fatty side is up and the rib side is on the bottom. Rub the seasoning onto the roast.

Step 3

Roast for 1 hour in the preheated oven. Turn the oven off and leave the roast inside. Do not open the door. Leave it in there for 3 hours. 30 to 40 minutes before serving, turn the oven back on at 375 degrees F (190 degrees C) to reheat the roast. The internal temperature should be at least 145 degrees F (62 degrees C). Remove from the oven and let rest for 10 minutes before carving into servings.

Nutrition Facts Per Serving:
576 calories; protein 37g 74% DV; carbohydrates 0.6g; fat 46.2g 71% DV; cholesterol 137.2mg 46% DV; sodium 879.6mg 35% DV.

SLOW ROASTED BBQ BEEF ROAST

Ingredients

5 pounds boneless rump roast

2 cloves garlic, sliced

1 teaspoon Spanish paprika

1 teaspoon salt

1 teaspoon pepper

¼ teaspoon dried rosemary

¼ teaspoon dried thyme

Directions

STEP 1

Prepare an outdoor rotisserie grill for medium heat.

STEP 2

Cut slits on all sides of the roast, and insert garlic slices.

STEP 3

In a small bowl, mix paprika, salt, pepper, rosemary, and thyme. Rub the mixture over the roast.

STEP 4

Place roast on the prepared rotisserie, and cook 2 to 5 hours, to a minimum internal temperature of 145 degrees F (63 degrees C). Allow to rest about 20 minutes before slicing.

Nutrition Facts Per Serving:

485 calories; protein 44.8g 90% DV; carbohydrates 0.5g; fat 32.5g 50% DV; cholesterol 138.3mg 46% DV; sodium 344mg 14% DV.

CAJUN ROAST BEEF

Ingredients

2 teaspoons garlic, minced

½ teaspoon prepared horseradish

1 teaspoon hot pepper sauce

1 teaspoon dried thyme

½ teaspoon salt

½ teaspoon ground black pepper

2 teaspoons Cajun seasoning

2 tablespoons olive oil

2 tablespoons malt vinegar

2 pounds beef eye of round roast

Directions

Step 1

Stir the garlic, horseradish, hot pepper sauce, thyme, salt, pepper, Cajun seasoning, olive oil, and malt vinegar together in a bowl until thoroughly blended.

Step 2

Pierce the beef roast all over with a meat fork. Place the roast in a large, resealable plastic bag. Spoon in the marinade and turn the roast so it's well coated. Refrigerate overnight, turning occasionally if desired.

Step 3

When ready to cook, place the roast in a slow cooker along with any remaining marinade. Do not add water. Roast on Low for 8 to 10 hours, or until desired doneness. For medium-rare, a meat thermometer should read 135 degrees F (57 degrees C). Remove from the slow cooker to a serving plate, and allow to rest 15 minutes before slicing across the grain.

Nutrition Facts Per Serving:

148 calories; protein 13.4g 27% DV; carbohydrates 1.1g; fat 9.7g 15% DV; cholesterol 35.6mg 12% DV; sodium 310.9mg 12% DV.

GRILLED TRI-TIP WITH OREGON HERB RUB

Ingredients

1 tablespoon salt

1 ½ teaspoons garlic salt

½ teaspoon celery salt

¼ teaspoon ground black pepper

¼ teaspoon onion powder

¼ teaspoon paprika

¼ teaspoon dried dill

¼ teaspoon dried sage

¼ teaspoon crushed dried rosemary

1 (2 1/2 pound) beef tri-tip roast

Directions

Step 1

Mix together the salt, garlic salt, celery salt, black pepper, onion powder, paprika, dill, sage, and rosemary in a bowl. Store in an airtight container at room temperature until ready to use.

Step 2

Use a damp towel to lightly moisten the roast with water, then pat with the prepared rub. Refrigerate for a minimum of 2 hours, up to overnight, for the flavors to fully come together.

Step 3

Preheat an outdoor grill for high heat and lightly oil grate.

Step 4

Place the roast onto the preheated grill and quickly cook until brown on all sides to sear the meat, then remove. Reset the grill for medium-low indirect heat (if using charcoal, move coals to the outside edges of the grill pit).

STEP 5

Return the roast to the grill, and cook, turning occasionally, until the desired degree of doneness has been reached, about 1 1/2 hours for medium-well. Remove from the grill and cover with aluminum foil. Allow to rest for 10 minutes before carving across the grain in thin slices to serve.

Nutrition Facts Per Serving:

214 calories; protein 30.4g 61% DV; carbohydrates 0.3g; fat 9.3g 14% DV; cholesterol 105.4mg 35% DV; sodium 1083.4mg 43% DV.

DYNAMITES

Ingredients

2 teaspoons vegetable oil

1 onion, chopped

2 pounds ground beef

4 eaches green bell peppers, chopped

1 (14.5 ounce) can diced tomatoes

1 (8 ounce) can tomato sauce

1 (6 ounce) can tomato paste

1 teaspoon crushed red pepper flakes

Directions

Step 1

Heat the oil in a saucepan over medium-high heat; cook the onion in the hot oil until tender, about 5 minutes. Add the ground beef, bell peppers, tomatoes, tomato sauce, tomato paste, and red pepper flakes to the saucepan; stir.

Step 2

Reduce heat to medium-low; simmer until the peppers are soft and the beef is tender, 4 to 6 hours.

Nutrition Facts Per Serving:

352 calories; protein 28.5g 57% DV; carbohydrates 15.3g

5% DV; fat 19.7g 30% DV; cholesterol 91.8mg 31% DV;
sodium 616.1mg 25% DV.

SPINACH AND FETA PITA BAKE

Ingredients

1 (6 ounce) tub sun-dried tomato pesto

6 (6 inch) whole wheat pita breads

2 plum tomato (blank)s roma (plum) tomatoes, chopped

1 bunch spinach, rinsed and chopped

4 medium (blank)s fresh mushrooms, sliced

½ cup crumbled feta cheese

2 tablespoons grated Parmesan cheese

3 tablespoons olive oil

Ground black pepper to taste

Directions

STEP 1

Preheat the oven to 350 degrees F (175 degrees C).

STEP 2

Spread tomato pesto onto one side of each pita bread and place them pesto-side up on a baking sheet. Top pitas with tomatoes, spinach, mushrooms, feta cheese, and Parmesan cheese; drizzle with olive oil and season with pepper.

Step 3
Bake in the preheated oven until pita breads are crisp, about 12 minutes. Cut pitas into quarters.

Nutrition Facts Per Serving:
350 calories; protein 11.6g 23% DV; carbohydrates 41.6g 13% DV; fat 17.1g 26% DV; cholesterol 12.6mg 4% DV; sodium 587.1mg 24% DV.

GREEK GOD PASTA

Ingredients

1 (16 ounce) package whole wheat rotini pasta

1 (16 ounce) can peeled and diced tomatoes, drained

2 tablespoons chopped green bell pepper

¼ cup chopped green onion

3 cups tomato sauce

1 teaspoon dried basil

1 teaspoon dried oregano

1 cup sliced black olives

½ cup shredded mozzarella cheese

2 tablespoons crumbled feta cheese

Directions
Step 1
Preheat the oven to 400 degrees F (200 degrees C).

STEP 2

Bring a large pot of lightly salted water to a boil. Add rotini pasta, and cook until al dente, about 8 minutes. Drain and pour into a deep casserole dish.

STEP 3

Stir tomatoes, green pepper, green onion, olives and tomato sauce into the pasta. Season with basil and oregano and mix until evenly blended. Sprinkle mozzarella and feta cheese over the top.

STEP 4

Bake for 30 minutes in the preheated oven, until cheese is melted and bubbly. Let stand for a few minutes before serving.

Nutrition Facts Per Serving:
371 calories; protein 16.4g 33% DV; carbohydrates 68.5g 22% DV; fat 6g 9% DV; cholesterol 8.8mg 3% DV; sodium 1068.1mg 43% DV.

SPINACH-FETA CASSEROLE

Ingredients

2 (10 ounce) packages frozen chopped spinach

8 ounces crumbled feta cheese

2 cups shredded mozzarella cheese

1 cup cubed processed cheese food

1 cup melted butter, divided

2 tablespoons distilled white vinegar

½ teaspoon garlic powder

Salt and pepper to taste

1 (16 ounce) package phyllo dough

Direction

STEP 1

Preheat oven to 425 degrees F (220 degrees C).

Step 2

In a large bowl, combine the spinach, feta cheese, mozzarella cheese, processed cheese food, 1/2 the butter, vinegar, garlic powder, salt and pepper. Mix well and set aside.

Step 3

Place a layer of phyllo dough into the bottom of a lightly greased 2-quart casserole dish. Spread the spinach and cheese mixture into the dish and top with 4 layers of phyllo dough, spraying each layer with butter-flavored cooking spray. Drizzle the remaining butter over the top.

Step 4

Bake at 425 degrees F (220 degrees C) for 20 minutes.

Nutrition Facts Per Serving:

548 calories; protein 18.6g 37% DV; carbohydrates 31.8g 10% DV; fat 37.7g 58% DV; cholesterol 108.4mg 36% DV; sodium 1164.1mg 47% DV.

A LOT MORE THAN PLAIN SPINACH PIE (GREEK BATSARIA)

Ingredients

3 large eggs eggs

1 pound chopped fresh spinach

3 leeks leeks, chopped

5 eaches green onions, chopped

2 ⅓ cups crumbled feta cheese

1 bunch parsley, chopped

1 bunch dill, chopped

1 bunch spearmint, chopped

1 teaspoon white sugar

1 cup milk

¾ cup olive oil

1 pinch salt and ground black pepper to taste

2 ½ cups all-purpose flour

½ cup semolina flour

1 pinch salt

¼ cup olive oil

2 cups water

1 ¼ cups grated Parmesan cheese

2 tablespoons cold butter, cut into pieces

2 tablespoons olive oil

Directions
Step 1
Preheat an oven to 350 degrees F (175 degrees C). Grease a deep 9x9 inch baking dish.

Step 2
Beat the eggs in a mixing bowl, then stir in the spinach, leeks, green onions, feta cheese, parsley, dill, spearmint, sugar, milk, and 3/4 cup of olive oil until evenly mixed. Season to taste with salt and pepper; set aside. Whisk together the all-purpose flour, semolina flour, and 1 pinch of salt in a mixing bowl. Stir in 1/4 cup of olive oil and the water until no lumps remain. Pour 2/3 of the batter into the prepared 9x9 inch pan, and spread out evenly. Spoon the spinach filling over the batter, then spoon the remaining batter overtop. Sprinkle with the Parmesan cheese, butter pieces, and 2 tablespoons of olive oil.

STEP 3

Bake in the preheated oven until the bottom crust and top has firmed and nicely browned, about 1 hour.

Nutrition Facts Per Serving:
650 calories; protein 20.1g 40% DV; carbohydrates 45g 15% DV; fat 44.1g 68% DV; cholesterol 115.3mg 38% DV; sodium 714.2mg 29% DV.

SPANAKOPITA

Ingredients

3 (10 ounce) packages frozen chopped spinach, thawed and drained

1 tablespoon vegetable oil

1 ½ cups finely chopped onion

8 ounces feta cheese, crumbled

1 ¼ cups shredded Swiss cheese

¾ cup grated Parmesan cheese

2 large eggs eggs, beaten

¼ cup chopped fresh parsley

1 dash ground cinnamon

1 cup butter, melted

1 (16 ounce) package phyllo dough

Directions

Step 1

Preheat oven to 375 degrees F (190 degrees C).

STEP 2

Place spinach in a steamer over 1 inch of boiling water, and cover. Cook until tender, about 2 to 6 minutes. Drain and press to remove all water. Meanwhile, heat oil in a large skillet over medium heat. Saute onion until tender, but do not brown. Stir in cooked spinach and continue cooking until all moisture has evaporated. Remove from heat and cool to room temperature.

Step 3

In a large bowl combine feta cheese, Swiss cheese, Parmesan cheese, eggs, parsley and cinnamon. Stir in spinach and onion mixture.

Step 4

Brush the bottom of a 17x11 inch jelly roll pan with butter. Place 1 sheet of dough in the bottom of the pan; brush with butter. Continue to layer 13 more sheets of dough, brushing every other sheet with butter. Spread spinach and cheese mixture over dough. Continue layering with remaining dough, brushing every other sheet with butter. Tuck edges of dough under. Brush top sheet with butter and, using a sharp knife, score top layer into diamonds.

Step 5

Bake in preheated oven for 40 minutes, or until golden brown.

Nutrition Facts Per Serving:

496 calories; protein 17.2g 35% DV; carbohydrates 31.1g 10% DV; fat 34.5g 53% DV; cholesterol 125.2mg 42% DV; sodium 816mg 33% DV.

JUICY ROASTED CHICKEN

Ingredients

1 (3 pound) whole chicken, giblets removed

Salt and black pepper to taste

1 tablespoon onion powder, or to taste

½ cup margarine, divided

1 stalk celery, leaves removed

Directions

Step 1

Preheat oven to 350 degrees F (175 degrees C).

Step 2

Place chicken in a roasting pan, and season generously inside and out with salt and pepper. Sprinkle inside and out with onion powder. Place 3 tablespoons margarine in the chicken cavity. Arrange dollops of the remaining margarine around the chicken's exterior. Cut the celery into 3 or 4 pieces, and place in the chicken cavity.

STEP 3

Bake uncovered 1 hour and 15 minutes in the preheated oven, to a minimum internal temperature of 180 degrees F (82 degrees C). Remove from heat, and baste with melted margarine and drippings. Cover with aluminum foil, and allow to rest about 30 minutes before serving.

Nutrition Facts Per Serving:
423 calories; protein 30.9g 62% DV; carbohydrates 1.2g; fat 32.1g 49% DV; cholesterol 97mg 32% DV; sodium 661.9mg 27% DV.

CRISPY ROASTED CHICKEN

Ingredients

1 teaspoon kosher salt

½ teaspoon caraway seeds

½ teaspoon dried sage

¼ teaspoon fennel seeds

¼ teaspoon coriander seeds

¼ teaspoon dried rosemary

2 tablespoons paprika

2 teaspoons garlic powder

2 teaspoons all-purpose flour

1 teaspoon onion powder

5 tablespoons vegetable oil

1 (4 pound) broiler-fryer chicken, cut in half lengthwise

Directions
Step 1
Preheat oven to 425 degrees F (220 degrees C).

Step 2
In a spice grinder or mortar, combine kosher salt, caraway

seeds, sage, fennel, coriander, and rosemary. Grind to a coarse powder. Transfer spice mixture to a bowl and stir in paprika, garlic powder, flour, and onion powder; mix in vegetable oil to make a smooth paste.

Step 3

Pat chicken halves dry with paper towels and tuck wing tips up behind the back. Brush spice paste onto chicken halves, coating both sides, taking care to season under wings and legs. Place chicken halves in baking dish or roasting pan with skin sides up, leaving space around chicken so halves aren't touching.

Step 4

Roast in preheated oven until a thermometer inserted in a thigh reads 165 degrees F (74 degrees C), about 1 hour. Remove from oven and let rest for 10 minutes before slicing.

Nutrition Facts Per Serving:

495 calories; protein 41.5g 83% DV; carbohydrates 3.1g 1% DV; fat 34.5g 53% DV; cholesterol 129.3mg 43% DV; sodium 445.6mg 18% DV.

GERMAN CHICKEN

Ingredients

4 skinless, boneless chicken breast halves

1 cup barbecue sauce

22 ounces sauerkraut

Directions

Step 1

Preheat oven to 350 degrees F (175 degrees C).

STEP 2

In a 9x13 inch baking dish, place the sauerkraut in a single layer. Place the chicken breasts on top of the sauerkraut. Pour the barbecue sauce over the chicken. Cover and bake in the preheated oven for 30 minutes or until the chicken is cooked and the juices run clear.

Nutrition Facts Per Serving:
253 calories; protein 28.6g 57% DV; carbohydrates 29.2g 9% DV; fat 1.9g 3% DV; cholesterol 68.4mg 23% DV; sodium 1794mg 72% DV.

ROAST DUCK WITH CHESTNUT STUFFING

Ingredients
Marinade:
1 onion, peeled and cut into chunks

1 parsley root, peeled and cut into chunks

1 carrot, roughly chopped

1 sprig fresh rosemary

2 bay leaves

1 teaspoon whole white peppercorns

2 cups dry white wine

1 whole duck

Stuffing:
2 cups finely chopped roasted chestnuts

1 apple, peeled and finely chopped

2 slices bread, diced

1 egg

1 teaspoon dried tarragon, or to taste

Salt and freshly ground pepper to taste

Wooden skewers

2 tablespoons rapeseed oil, or more if needed

Directions

STEP 1

Combine onion, parsley root, carrot, rosemary, bay leaves, and white peppercorns in a bowl. Stir in white wine. Place duck in a large bowl and pour marinade over duck. Cover with foil and marinate in the fridge for at least 12 hours.

STEP 2

Preheat oven to 425 degrees F (220 degrees C).

STEP 3

Combine chestnuts, apple, bread, and egg in a bowl; season with tarragon, salt, and pepper.

STEP 4

Remove duck from the marinade and strain marinade through a sieve. Dry duck inside and out with paper towels. Rub salt and pepper all over the skin. Fill cavity with stuffing, being careful not to overstuff. Secure opening with wooden skewers. Pour oil into a roasting dish. Add stuffed duck, breast-side up.

STEP 5

Roast duck in the preheated oven, turning occasionally, until golden brown on all sides, about 20 minutes.

STEP 6

Heat marinade in a saucepan over medium heat until warmed through, about 5 minutes.

STEP 7

Pour warm marinade into the roasting pan. Cover with a lid or aluminum foil and return to the oven. Reduce oven temperature to 350 degrees F (175 degrees C) and bake duck until no longer pink at the bone and the juices run clear, about 90 minutes. An instant-read thermometer inserted into the thickest part of the thigh, near the bone, should read 165 degrees F (74 degrees C).

Step 8

Remove duck from the roasting pan and transfer to a baking sheet. Set oven rack about 6 inches from the heat source and preheat the oven's broiler. Roast duck until skin is golden-brown, 3 to 5 minutes. Remove duck from the oven, cover with a doubled sheet of aluminum foil, and allow to rest in a warm area for 10 minutes before slicing.

Step 9

Strain the stock, removing any burnt bits and skimming off fat. Heat stock in a saucepan over high heat and cook until gravy is reduced to 1/3, 5 to 10 minutes. Season with salt and pepper. Carve duck and serve with gravy.

Nutrition Facts Per Serving:

302 calories; protein 7.2g 14% DV; carbohydrates 36g 12% DV; fat 8g 12% DV; cholesterol 47.2mg 16% DV; sodium 132.1mg 5% DV.

GRILLHAXE (GRILLED EISBEIN, PORK SHANKS)

Ingredients

1 cup olive oil

2 tablespoons dried marjoram

2 tablespoons dried basil

2 tablespoons chopped fresh thyme

2 tablespoons chopped fresh rosemary

2 tablespoons sea salt

1 teaspoon paprika

1 teaspoon ground black pepper

1 teaspoon vegetable bouillon powder

6 (1 1/2) pounds pork shanks

Directions

Step 1

Preheat oven to 350 degrees F (175 degrees C).

Step 2

Whisk olive oil, marjoram, basil, rosemary, thyme, sea

salt, paprika, black pepper, and vegetable bouillon powder together in a bowl. Rub pork shanks with herb rub and arrange on a large baking pan.

STEP 3

Roast in preheated oven until shanks are tender and outer skin is crispy, about 3 hours.

Nutrition Facts Per Serving:
532 calories; protein 70.6g 141% DV; carbohydrates 0.8g; fat 27.9g 43% DV; cholesterol 185.9mg 62% DV; sodium 3080.5mg 123% DV.

HOMEMADE CHORIZO

Ingredients

1 clove garlic

3 teaspoons dried oregano

½ cup distilled white vinegar

½ cup crushed red pepper flakes

½ cup water

2½ pounds ground pork

Directions
Step 1
In a blender, combine garlic, oregano, vinegar, red pepper flakes, and water. Blend until smooth.

STEP 2

In a bowl pour mixture over ground pork; cover and refrigerate all day. Pour off any water that accumulates. Refrigerate or freeze for future use.

Nutrition Facts Per Serving:
322 calories; protein 26.3g 53% DV; carbohydrates 5.5g 2% DV; fat 21.9g 34% DV; cholesterol 92mg 31% DV; sodium 74.7mg 3% DV.

CONCLUSION

Tick numbers have been correlated quite well with cases of Lyme disease in most studies, and there is good evidence that tick numbers have increased recently as a result of climate change. Climate change has led to increased tick lifespans, increased migration of tick-carrying animals, and human development of wild areas where the ticks reside. All these factors potentially increase human exposure to tick bites. Having an optimal diet to minimize the inflammation that affects people with Lyme disease is very important. This is not so much aimed at eliminating the bacteria that cause Lyme disease as making it easier to live with Lyme disease by reducing symptoms. It may also help you respond better to any antibiotics you take.

www.ingramcontent.com/pod-product-compliance
Lightning Source LLC
Chambersburg PA
CBHW071532150726
48000CB00002B/780